ONE DAY AT A TIME

2021 DIARY

A Year-Long Journey of Personal Healing and Transformation

Abby Wynne

GILL BOOKS

Gill Books

Hume Avenue

Park West

Dublin 12

www.gillbooks.ie

Gill Book is an imprint of M.H. Gill and Co.

© Abby Wynne 2020

978 0 7171 8946 5

All photographs courtesy Unsplash.

Designed by Jane Matthews

Printed by BZ Graf, Poland

This book is typeset in Neutraface.

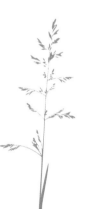

The paper used in this book comes from the wood pulp

of managed forests. For every tree felled, at least one

tree is planted, thereby renewing natural resources.

A CIP catalogue record for this book is available from the British Library.

5 4 3 2 1

What you hold inside of you is reflected
outwards and ripples into the world.
The times we are in call us to step into
the truth of who we are and leave behind
our timidness and inauthenticity.

For those who are brave enough to step up
to this challenge, I dedicate this diary –
and all the healing in it – to you.

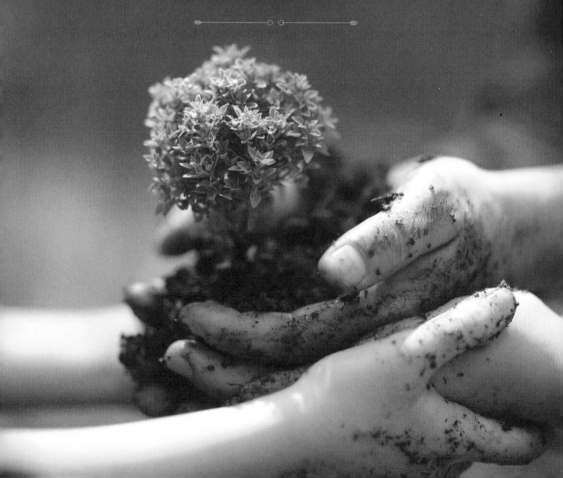

ABOUT THE AUTHOR

Abby Wynne is a healer and author who blends shamanism, psychotherapy and energy healing in a powerful way that creates lasting change. She is the bestselling author of many books, including *Planting the Seeds: Poetry, Stories and Prayers*, *The Book of Healing Affirmations*, *How to Be Well* and *Heal your Inner Wounds*. Her passion is teaching people how to look after their spiritual, emotional and mental health so that they can create vibrant and happy lives for themselves.

Abby's core teachings work towards empowering you to do your inner work with strength and courage while providing a structure and foundation to guide you. Her healing practice has many clients from around the world, and Abby's Online Academy website offers self-paced and group-led online programmes in which you can participate from the comfort of your own home. Abby also facilitates monthly group healing sessions, where everyone is welcome, and a healing circle with membership benefits.

Abby lives in Ireland with her husband, four children and dog, Milo.
You can join Abby on Facebook at Abby's Energy Healing Page,
Instagram @abbynrghealing, Twitter @abbynrghealing or connect with her
through her website, www.abby-wynne.com.

Abby has made special downloadable files to go with this diary to
enhance your healing experience. They are free, and you can find them
on her website, www.abby-wynne.com/onedayatatime.

'An awake heart is like a sky that pours light.'

Hafez

Name

Address

Telephone

Emergency contact

USEFUL DATES

January

Friday 1st ....New Year's Day

February

Monday 1st...St Brigid's Day

March

Wednesday 17th ....St Patrick's Day National Holiday

Saturday 20th ....Spring Equinox

April

Monday 5th...Easter National Holiday

May

Monday 3rd...May Public Holiday

June

Monday 7th...June Public Holiday

Monday 21st...Summer Solstice

August

Monday 2nd...August Public Holiday

September

Wednesday 22nd ....Autumn Equinox

October

Monday 25th...October Public Holiday

December

Tuesday 21st...Winter Solstice

Saturday 25th...Christmas Day

Sunday 26th...St Stephen's Day

Friday 31st...New Year's Eve

THEMES FOR THIS YEAR

January...Compassion and Self-Care

February ....Freedom and Joy

March ....Expansion and Growth

April ....Inspiration and Creativity

May...Purification and Healing

June ....Peace and Forgiveness

July...Authenticity and Vitality

August...Presence and Beauty

September...Safety and Grounding

October ....Balance and Stability

November ....Resilience and Grace

December ....Love and Gratitude

MOON PHASES CALENDAR
2021

January	6 ◑	13 ●	20 ◐	28 ○	
February	4 ◑	11 ●	19 ◐	27 ○	
March	6 ◑	13 ●	21 ◐	28 ○	
April	4 ◑	12 ●	20 ◐	27 ○	
May	3 ◑	11 ●	19 ◐	26 ○	
June	2 ◑	10 ●	18 ◐	24 ○	
July	1 ◑	10 ●	17 ◐	24 ○	31 ◑
August	8 ●	15 ◐	22 ○	30 ◑	
September	7 ●	13 ◐	21 ○	29 ◑	
October	6 ●	13 ◐	20 ○	28 ◑	
November	4 ●	11 ◐	19 ○	27 ◑	
December	4 ●	11 ◐	19 ○	27 ◑	

SPECIAL MOON EVENTS
2021

| **Thursday 10 June** | Solar Eclipse |
| **Thursday 18 November** | Lunar Eclipse |

CALENDAR
2021

JANUARY

Su	Mo	Tu	We	Th	Fr	Sa
					1	2
3	4	5	6	7	8	9
10	11	12	13	14	15	16
17	18	19	20	21	22	23
24	25	26	27	28	29	30
31						

FEBRUARY

Su	Mo	Tu	We	Th	Fr	Sa
	1	2	3	4	5	6
7	8	9	10	11	12	13
14	15	16	17	18	19	20
21	22	23	24	25	26	27
28						

MARCH

Su	Mo	Tu	We	Th	Fr	Sa
	1	2	3	4	5	6
7	8	9	10	11	12	13
14	15	16	17	18	19	20
21	22	23	24	25	26	27
28	29	30	31			

APRIL

Su	Mo	Tu	We	Th	Fr	Sa
				1	2	3
4	5	6	7	8	9	10
11	12	13	14	15	16	17
18	19	20	21	22	23	24
25	26	27	28	29	30	

MAY

Su	Mo	Tu	We	Th	Fr	Sa
						1
2	3	4	5	6	7	8
9	10	11	12	13	14	15
16	17	18	19	20	21	22
23	24	25	26	27	28	29
30	31					

JUNE

Su	Mo	Tu	We	Th	Fr	Sa
	1	2	3	4	5	
6	7	8	9	10	11	12
13	14	15	16	17	18	19
20	21	22	23	24	25	26
27	28	29	30			

JULY

Su	Mo	Tu	We	Th	Fr	Sa
				1	2	3
4	5	6	7	8	9	10
11	12	13	14	15	16	17
18	19	20	21	22	23	24
25	26	27	28	29	30	31

AUGUST

Su	Mo	Tu	We	Th	Fr	Sa
1	2	3	4	5	6	7
8	9	10	11	12	13	14
15	16	17	18	19	20	21
22	23	24	25	26	27	28
29	30	31				

SEPTEMBER

Su	Mo	Tu	We	Th	Fr	Sa
			1	2	3	4
5	6	7	8	9	10	11
12	13	14	15	16	17	18
19	20	21	22	23	24	25
26	27	28	29	30		

OCTOBER

Su	Mo	Tu	We	Th	Fr	Sa
					1	2
3	4	5	6	7	8	9
10	11	12	13	14	15	16
17	18	19	20	21	22	23
24	25	26	27	28	29	30
31						

NOVEMBER

Su	Mo	Tu	We	Th	Fr	Sa
	1	2	3	4	5	6
7	8	9	10	11	12	13
14	15	16	17	18	19	20
21	22	23	24	25	26	27
28	23	30				

DECEMBER

Su	Mo	Tu	We	Th	Fr	Sa
			1	2	3	4
5	6	7	8	9	10	11
12	13	14	15	16	17	18
19	20	21	22	23	24	25
26	27	28	29	30	31	

HOW TO USE THIS DIARY

There are several ways to use this diary; however you choose to use it is up to you. You can enjoy the flow of the graphics, the energy of the affirmations and quotes, and use the spaces to write down your appointments and to-do lists. Or you can use the energy of each month to inspire you and the writing space for journaling your thoughts and emotions. Think of this diary as a friend who reminds you to be nicer to yourself, encouraging you to take some time out for you.

This diary is designed to support you through the energy shifts of the coming year, through the monthly themes, exercises, affirmations and ways for you to go deeper. Again, it is up to you whether you spend time with this or not. Anything goes – there are no rules. I have written everything except for the 'going deeper' suggestions in the present tense to help bring you more into the present moment – this is a way to slow down, step out of time and reconnect to your heart. The more familiar you are with the words I use and the more you believe them to be true for you as you read them, the deeper the impact they will have on your healing process.

The basic premise of all my work is this: The relationship you have with yourself is the foundation of all your relationships. When you're kind to yourself, compassionate and at peace, you have a much more wholehearted life. Take it one day at a time – that's all any of us can do.

Blessings to you on your healing journey this year.

THEMES

This diary will be able to travel with you through the ebbs and flows of emotional energy that you may experience as you move through the year. I have consulted with Lorna Bevan, of Hare in the Moon Astrology, and have designed the themes around the coming astrological shifts, so that the diary will support you when times are difficult and enhance your ability for healing and growth wherever possible.

Try to take time at the beginning of each month to connect to that month's theme. Make time during the month to do the exercises. If you feel yourself coming out of balance, come back to the monthly invocation and reconnect. Reading the words out loud is much more powerful than reading them quietly to yourself. The affirmations are more powerful when you feel them deeply in your body, rather than just saying the words. They can help bring you back into balance if you're feeling off-centre. You can also replay the downloadable materials as often as you wish, as additional support to help you feel grounded.

We are all different. We flow and change with time. One month you may delve deep, and another you may not – that's OK. If you choose to do the work that is offered here, to do it wholeheartedly you must do it your own way. Feel into it and you will know what is right for you. As time goes on, you will become more confident. A year is a long time, but it passes very quickly too.

At the end of each month, you are invited to reflect on how the month's theme impacted upon you. It's a way for you to mark the occasion and, over time, is a good record of how far you have come on your healing journey. Using this diary gives you an opportunity to create, to dream and to grow, while tracking your progress throughout the year.

AFFIRMATIONS

Affirmations are statements of great meaning. I see them as a very powerful tool of transformation, if used with strong intention behind them. If you simply say an affirmation out loud by reading it, there is no power in it because you are just reading a group of words. If you take some time, however, to bring your presence inwards and feel into the meaning and power behind each word in the affirmation, then the energy behind the affirmation changes, and it can change your energy too.

Being in alignment with an affirmation happens when your mind, your heart and your gut instinct all resonate with it. For example, 'I deserve to be happy' could be something your mind agrees with, but there may be a hidden belief somewhere in you that doesn't agree at all. This belief can keep sabotaging you, just when things seem to be going well in your life. Saying 'I deserve to be happy' without the depth of feeling is a lost opportunity for you to learn if you are actually in alignment with it or not. Learning that you're not in alignment is a great opportunity to heal the part of you that doesn't believe, so that you can transform it and it no longer remains an obstacle in your life.

Try this exercise – choose an affirmation out of the book right now. Open the diary at any page and see which affirmation jumps out at you. Read the words silently to yourself, then bring your awareness inwards. Now speak the affirmation out loud with emotion. Does it sound like you believe it? Say it again and notice what you're thinking. If the mind believes it, you'll be fine with it, but if it doesn't, you'll hear all the reasons why it's not true for you. That's great! This is about getting to know yourself better.

Now say it again, only say it from your heart. Ask your heart whether it totally agrees with what you have just said. Listen to your emotional response – are you soft and open, or are have you shut down? Say it again one more time with your awareness in your stomach and your gut. Do you feel strong, peaceful and stable, or do you feel nervous, anxious and ungrounded?

There are no right or wrong answers – what is true for you is your truth, but sometimes our truth is based on old things we learned as children that are no longer valid for us as adults. Examining what you hold as truth is part of a healing process so that you can decide if it still is a truth for you, or if it's something you would like to do some work on.

The affirmations in this diary are not daily; in fact, most of them span several days This is to give you time to really tune in to them so you can learn which ones you are not in alignment with and take the time to become so if you wish to. Try to say the affirmations each day, several times a day, with meaning, and let them grow on you.

Healing is not about forcing or pushing change but creating a space for you to grow. You're already perfect as you are, and if you don't believe that, perhaps that's an affirmation you'd like to work with too.

EXERCISES

The exercises are designed to help you relax and come more into the moment, and to help you find balance and stability. Try each one more than once. As you settle into them and get used to the feeling of being more in the moment, you may find them more effective for you. Try the free audio downloads from my website if you are having trouble settling. Let my voice create a safe space for you where you can really let go and relax. You can put the audio files on your mobile device and then you can listen to them anyplace, anywhere, for a ten-minute mindfulness break.

GOING DEEPER

Thinking, writing and visualising are all part of healing, but so is taking action. I have given you ways to go deeper with the healing work for each month, but you don't have to do any of them. If you have a different idea that suits you better, do that instead!

CHECKING IN

Every three months I will ask you to take some time out to contemplate what you've just been experiencing, so that you can come into alignment with it and recognise the learning you've received. This is an optional activity, but it will deepen your experience of growth and healing with this diary.

WHAT TO WRITE

I totally understand that brand new, beautifully crisp, clean pages can be off-putting when it comes to putting pen to paper. However, this is your diary, and that is what it is here for. You don't need to pressure yourself to get it perfect, and you don't need to write for an audience either. All you need to do is write a thought or a feeling, make a list, or keep track of your emotions. Fun ideas include using different-coloured pens, doodling with colouring pencils, or even writing how you feel in poetry. So smudge away, cross out stuff and mess up that pretty page, but get the words out there. Once you get started, the writing will flow.

It might help if you take a minute or two to slow down and bring your awareness inwards before you start your writing. Perhaps take some time to breathe and disconnect from whatever is pulling you out of the present moment. Use the space to write down what is distracting you, so you can tell your mind, 'Look, I know, and

I've written it down! So you can stop reminding me!' You could ask yourself 'What do I need to know today?' and then listen to your inner wisdom and write that down, as if you're taking dictation from a wise friend who is speaking to you. You could also write down what went well for you that day and what didn't, so you can remember what you would prefer to do the next time.

You could also rewrite the affirmation for the day or write a new one where one isn't present. Use the diary to write about what you need to do to look after you, or simply write in your appointments and your plans.

If you want, you can use the following prompts and see where they lead you: Today I feel ... Today I know ... Today I believe ... Today I am ... Today I want ... Today I wish ...

You've got a whole year ahead of you, and lots of ideas and opportunities. Try them all, or only a few. Above all, please be patient with yourself. It's all here for you, so take your time and use this diary in a way that feels right for you.

SETTING YOUR INTENTION

Setting an intention for the year is a very powerful thing to do. Some people like to choose a single word for the year as a general theme, such as empowerment, joy, connection or growth. I like to make it a little more specific by writing down a statement or a paragraph that I can come back to time and time again. The beauty of setting an intention is that it can change and grow as you change and grow. The power behind it comes with your awareness of it.

Here's an example of an intention for the year that you can use, but it is better if you write one yourself.

This year I will go easier on myself and let my heart and soul lead me on my journey of healing and growth. I am beginning to see how I'm already enough, just as I am. I want to make a commitment to let go of my expectations I put on myself, and allow myself to just be who I am, instead of forcing or pushing myself to be something else.

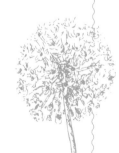

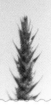

My intention for my healing journey for 2021:

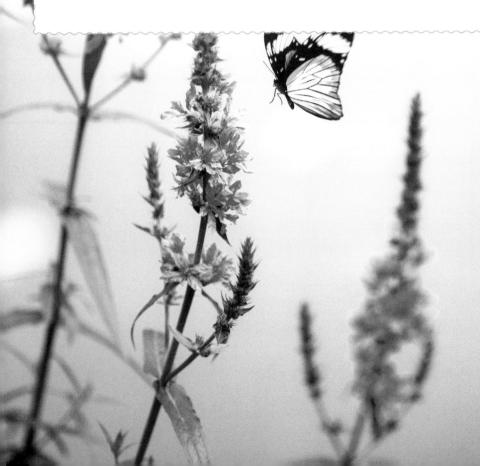

COMPASSION AND SELF-CARE

**For I respond best to love,
as love is what truly heals.**

'It's not selfish to love yourself, take care of yourself,
and make your happiness a priority. It's necessary.'

Mandy Hale

JANUARY

I start into the new year gently, realising that too much change too quickly never sticks. My resolution this year is simply to learn how to love myself more. I've always been afraid to do this because it means I actually have to show up and take responsibility for myself. I know that if I don't look after myself, I will grow resentful of those who I expect to do it for me. The quality of my life is up to me. I really do want it to improve. Perhaps all I need do, to tip the balance in my favour, is be more compassionate to myself. This month I resolve to be nicer to myself, to give myself space to grow, and to not push or force or try to fix. Instead, I will be kind, patient and caring. By being compassionate and generous to me, I fill myself up and meet my own needs. This frees me up to be happy.

EXERCISE

I open my eyes slowly and look at my reflection in the mirror. Do I recognise and accept myself completely? I stand and stay soft with myself until I see myself at a deeper level – the scars, the lines and how I am ageing. I see my experiences written on my face. I honour and accept that I did the best I could with what I knew at the time. I soften and open my heart to myself and all that I have gone through in my life. I can say wholeheartedly that it is good to be me.

GOING DEEPER

What else would you like to say to yourself? Have a conversation with yourself as you look in the mirror. Listen to what you need as you say it back to yourself. Resolve that this month you will set your intention to putting your self-care plan into action, however difficult it may seem. Do something nice for yourself: take long walks or hot baths, treat yourself to beautiful body oils and perfumed creams. Have a delicious hair treatment, all while staying focused in your heart.

FRIDAY 1

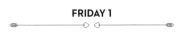

I am learning how to love all the parts of me

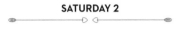

SATURDAY 2

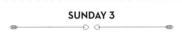

SUNDAY 3

I accept myself just as I am in this moment

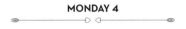

MONDAY 4

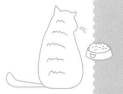

TUESDAY 5

Self-care means looking after myself better

WEDNESDAY 6

I do not need to fix or change anyone else

THURSDAY 7

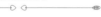

I let go of the pressure that I put on myself

FRIDAY 8

Love softens all of my sharp edges

SATURDAY 9

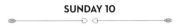

I take responsibility for my own self-care

SUNDAY 10

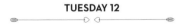

I slow down and bring myself into the present moment

MONDAY 11

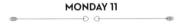

I am able to look after myself

TUESDAY 12

WEDNESDAY 13

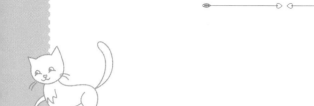

I no longer need to get tangled up to please someone else

THURSDAY 14

I send love and compassion to all aspects of me, even the ones I have difficulty with

FRIDAY 15

SATURDAY 16

I move through the day with compassion and love

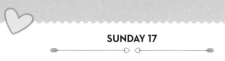

SUNDAY 17

Giving myself what I need is self-care

MONDAY 18

TUESDAY 19

I see myself and all that I have experienced, and I appreciate how far I have come

WEDNESDAY 20

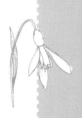

I give myself permission to take some time for me today

THURSDAY 21

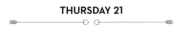

When I am kind to myself, I have more kindness to offer other people

FRIDAY 22

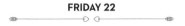

I disconnect from fear and anger and I choose kindness and love

SATURDAY 23

I release myself from my expectations of myself

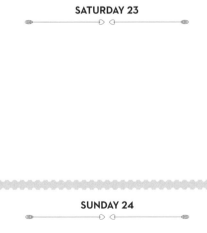

SUNDAY 24

I release myself from my expectations of myself

MONDAY 25

I am good enough just as I am

TUESDAY 26

I don't need to compare myself to anyone else

WEDNESDAY 27

I allow myself to make mistakes and learn from them

THURSDAY 28

I am learning how to give myself more of the things that I enjoy

FRIDAY 29

I give other people the freedom that I also give to myself

SATURDAY 30

I let go of my need to control the situation

SUNDAY 31

I feel safe to experience all of my emotions

NOTES ON COMPASSION AND SELF-CARE

WHAT IS DIFFICULT FOR YOU WHEN IT COMES TO SELF-CARE? SPEND SOME TIME FINDING OUT WHAT YOUR CORE BELIEF IS AROUND LOOKING AFTER YOURSELF. DECIDE IF IT IS A HEALTHY BELIEF OR NOT.

COMPASSION FOR YOURSELF GIVES YOU SOME SPACE TO BREATHE, AND WHEN YOU HAVE THIS SPACE YOU HAVE MORE SPACE FOR OTHERS. WHAT ABOUT THIS STATEMENT CAUSES YOU DIFFICULTY? CAN YOU SEE A CONNECTION BETWEEN THIS AND YOUR CORE BELIEF AROUND SELF-CARE? WHAT WOULD YOU LIKE TO CHANGE ABOUT IT?

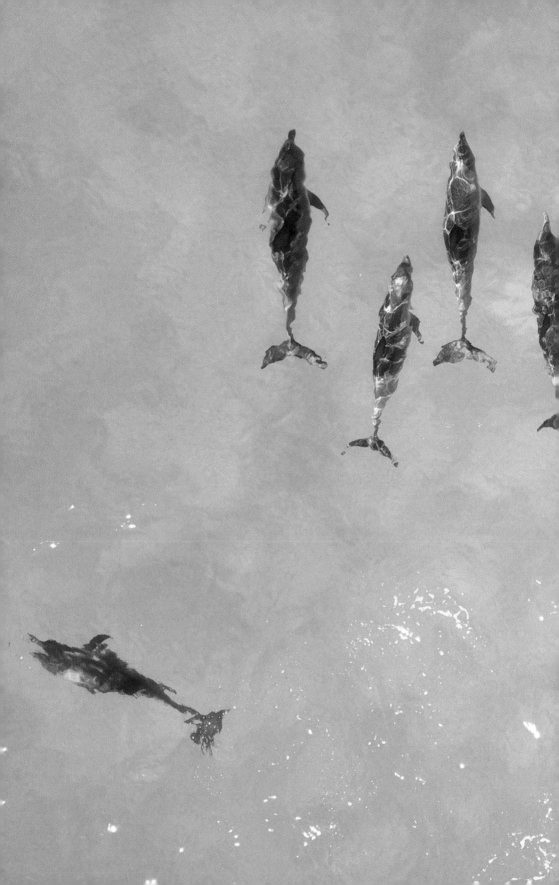

FEBRUARY

FREEDOM AND JOY

Joy will not knock me over when I am unbound from the heaviness of my life.

'Love is a by-product of freedom; it is the overflowing joy of freedom, it is the fragrance of freedom. First the freedom has to be there, then love follows.'

Osho

FEBRUARY

Learning how to look after myself better has freed me up from my expectations of others. I now allow myself to expand and take up my full space in the world. I have nothing to apologise for. I am human. I make mistakes, just as we all do. I'm learning how to be my best self and I'm doing okay. This month I'm inviting joy into my life, for it is beautiful to be alive. I want to allow myself to truly feel the wonder of nature, the beauty of love and the capacity that I hold to be happy. I know that life will not wait for me to catch up with it, and that my life is never going to be fully the way I want it to be. I free myself from my need for everything to be perfect. I give myself permission to be joyful, and to deliberately spend time doing the things I love.

EXERCISE

I see myself on a clifftop overlooking the sea. The sun shines down on me and melts all of my emotional pain and burdens. I feel lighter. The wind blows through me and clears away any energy I have picked up from other people. I am allowed to be happy. I jump into the sky and dive down into the water. Just as I enter it, I become a dolphin. Beauty and joy fills my heart. I swim fast and free through the crystal waters. They heal me. It feels like flying. I am free.

GOING DEEPER

Plant some bulbs or seeds in your garden or in a pot. Spend some time with them every day. Know that when you cannot see the growth, it doesn't mean it isn't happening. Get to know the plant. Watch it as it grows, unfolds and blossoms. It knows what to do, and so do you. After your time with the plant, ask yourself what you need to do for yourself, and then do it.

MONDAY 1

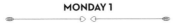

I deliberately invite joy into my life

TUESDAY 2

WEDNESDAY 3

I choose to focus on lightness and joy today

THURSDAY 4

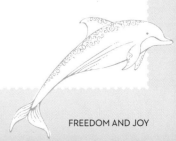

I do not need to live in fear anymore

FREEDOM AND JOY

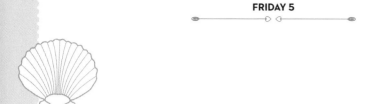

FRIDAY 5

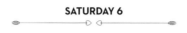

I give myself permission to be myself completely

SATURDAY 6

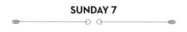

I disconnect from heaviness and reconnect to a source of joy

SUNDAY 7

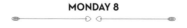

I take time to slow down and bring my awareness back to my centre

MONDAY 8

I can be serious, joyful and free all at the same time

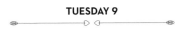

TUESDAY 9

I send long, deep roots from my feet into Mother Earth and I am held

WEDNESDAY 10

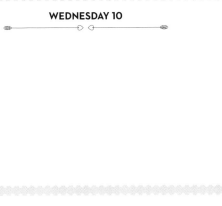

THURSDAY 11

I can open my wings and unfold to my true size no matter where I am

FRIDAY 12

It is safe to open my heart to joy

SATURDAY 13

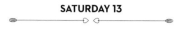

I no longer need to carry heavy energies

SUNDAY 14

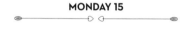

I let go of all that keeps me from experiencing joy

MONDAY 15

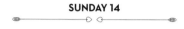

Today I will pay attention to the good things that are going on around me

TUESDAY 16

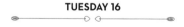

I am grateful for the synchronicities and messages that I receive from the Universe

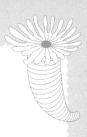

WEDNESDAY 17

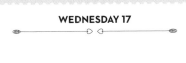

THURSDAY 18

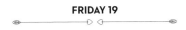

I take time to sit in stillness and breathe and come back to my centre

FRIDAY 19

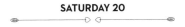

I can listen to everybody's opinion and then decide for myself

SATURDAY 20

I allow myself to experience all of my emotions

SUNDAY 21

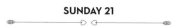

When I am joyful, I shine my light a little brighter

MONDAY 22

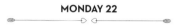

I can find the beauty in small things

TUESDAY 23

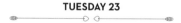

I choose to resonate with the energy of freedom and joy

WEDNESDAY 24

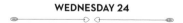

I open my heart to joy and let more joy come through me and into the world

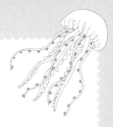

THURSDAY 25

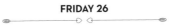

I can spend time doing the things I love without guilt

FRIDAY 26

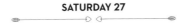

I give myself permission to express myself

SATURDAY 27

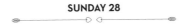

I don't need to have all the answers today

SUNDAY 28

I feel the joy and freedom that comes from knowing who I am

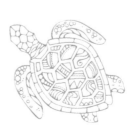

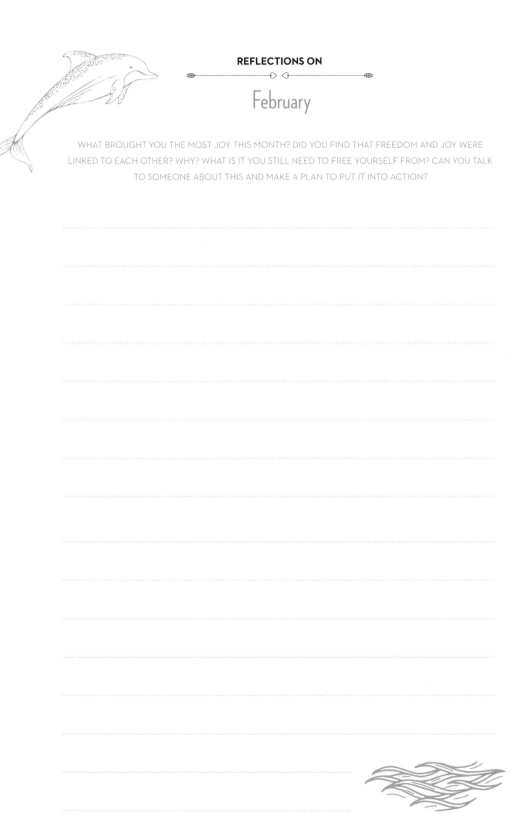

REFLECTIONS ON

February

WHAT BROUGHT YOU THE MOST JOY THIS MONTH? DID YOU FIND THAT FREEDOM AND JOY WERE LINKED TO EACH OTHER? WHY? WHAT IS IT YOU STILL NEED TO FREE YOURSELF FROM? CAN YOU TALK TO SOMEONE ABOUT THIS AND MAKE A PLAN TO PUT IT INTO ACTION?

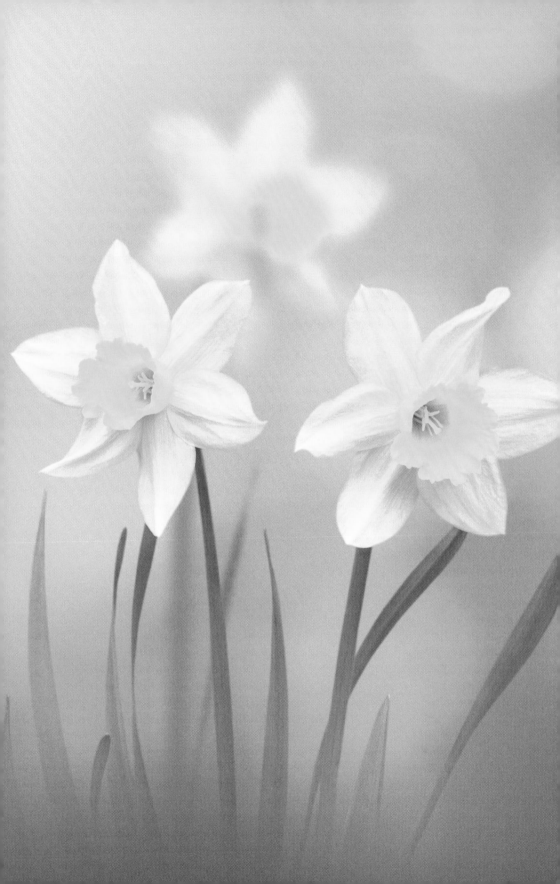

EXPANSION AND GROWTH

Like the caterpillar wraps itself into a cocoon not really knowing why, I'll follow my instinct.

'The shell must break before the bird can fly.'

Alfred Tennyson

MARCH

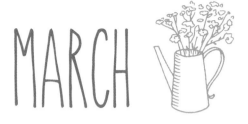

This month I'll trust the process of healing and look after me. I know growth can be painful. I may need to take more time alone, and I offer that space to myself. I pledge to listen to my inner voice, say no when my body says no, and only take on as much as I am able. Drawing from my renewed source of self-compassion, I will be patient as I shed my skin, I will be kind to myself as I go inwards, and I will trust that I shall emerge stronger, wiser, and the better for it. I am grateful for the heat that turns the coal into the diamond, for it is in the richness and beauty of diamond light that we can truly appreciate the wonder of the world. I am the coal. I am the diamond. I allow this process of expansion and growth so that I can shine my diamond light brighter and stronger out into the world, to where it is needed the most.

EXERCISE

I can hear my breath. I slow down and feel my feet on the ground. I breathe – one, two, three – and with each breath I feel softer, lighter and more connected to me. I imagine a diamond light shining out from my heart centre. As I focus on it, with each breath, it gets stronger and bigger until it fills my whole body and shines outwards into the world.

GOING DEEPER

Spend time every day slowing down, coming back into your body, and attending to your own needs. These needs can change depending on how you are feeling, so really take the time to get to know your likes and dislikes. Let go of the things that you do because you feel you should do them, if they are not truly beneficial to you.

MONDAY 1

I let go of my idea of who I should be and allow myself to be who I am

TUESDAY 2

WEDNESDAY 3

I take the time that I need to do the things I need to do

THURSDAY 4

I slow down and listen to my breath

FRIDAY 5

I disconnect from other people's drama and choose to be at peace in my heart

SATURDAY 6

SUNDAY 7

I am learning how to make healthy choices

MONDAY 8

I respect all human beings no matter where they are on their journey

TUESDAY 9

WEDNESDAY 10

I no longer need to fix or change anything

THURSDAY 11

I give myself all the time I need to grow and heal

FRIDAY 12

I expand my light out into the world and feel at peace

SATURDAY 13

SUNDAY 14

I feel safe to experience all of my emotions

MONDAY 15

The ground is beneath me, the sky is above me, I feel held

TUESDAY 16

I am patient and kind with myself

WEDNESDAY 17

My day begins and ends with peace

THURSDAY 18

I am compassionate and kind with myself and others

FRIDAY 19

SATURDAY 20

I have good, strong, energetic boundaries

SUNDAY 21
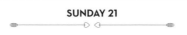

I completely accept myself just as I am

MONDAY 22
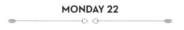

Every experience is an opportunity for learning

TUESDAY 23
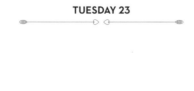

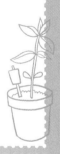

WEDNESDAY 24

What I want and what I need are not always the same thing

THURSDAY 25

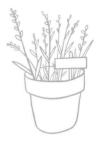

Today I make all my choices from a place of love

FRIDAY 26

I slow down and bring my awareness into the present moment

SATURDAY 27

I open my heart and shine my light out to the world

SUNDAY 28

I let go of the pressure that I put on myself to be perfect

MONDAY 29

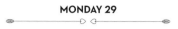

I choose love, compassion and understanding

TUESDAY 30

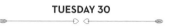

I surround myself with people and things that fill me with love

WEDNESDAY 31

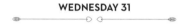

I am worthy, and I am enough just as I am

NOTES ON EXPANSION AND GROWTH

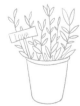

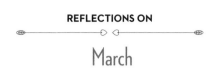

March

WHAT WAS THE HARDEST PART OF THIS MONTH AND WHY? WHAT WAS YOUR BIGGEST LEARNING?
WHAT WOULD YOU LIKE TO INVITE INTO YOUR LIFE NEXT MONTH?

CHECKING IN

The themes for the first part of the year were
Compassion and Self-Care, Freedom and Joy,
Expansion and Growth.

Take some time right now to sit with all that you have learned
and all that you feel you have achieved.
Well done.

WHAT DO YOU FEEL WAS YOUR GREATEST MOMENT OF THE PAST THREE MONTHS?

WHAT WAS THE MOST DIFFICULT? HOW DID YOU LOOK AFTER YOURSELF IN IT?

GO BACK THROUGH THE DIARY AND CHOOSE YOUR FAVOURITE AFFIRMATION,
THE ONE FROM THE PAST THREE MONTHS THAT MADE THE MOST DIFFERENCE TO YOU.
WRITE IT DOWN HERE FOR SAFEKEEPING.

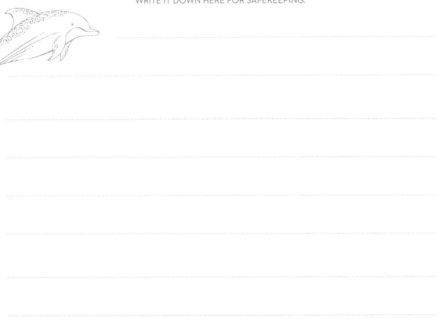

Go to my website, www.abby-wynne.com/onedayatatime, and make sure you have signed
up for my bonus recordings. Perhaps you'd like to take some time to listen to a few of the
visualisations and meditations to consolidate what you have done so far this year.

Now we move to the next three months of the year. Don't forget you can revisit
any of the affirmations and exercises from the past three months and bring them with
you as additional support.

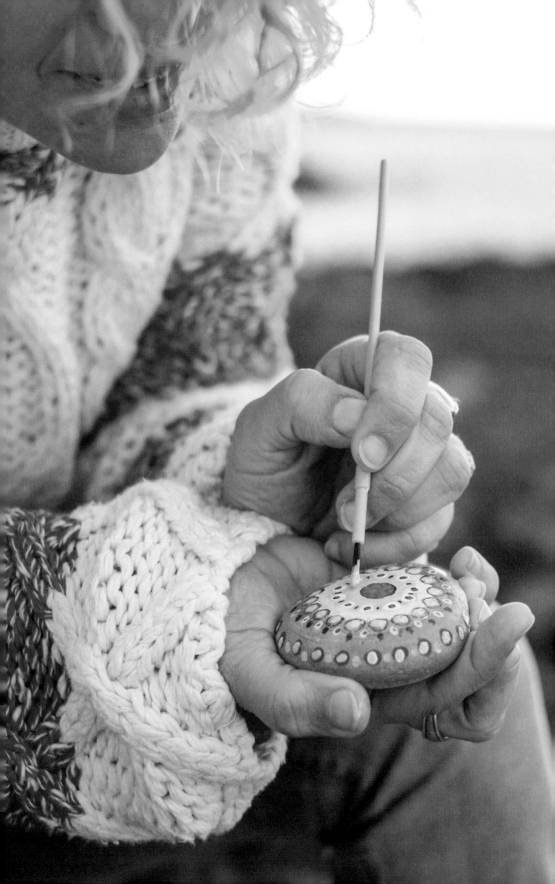

INSPIRATION AND CREATIVITY

My Soul longs to sing, dance, paint and write.
I will make the space to create, for if not now,
then when?

'Our wounds are often the openings into the best
and most beautiful part of us.'

David Richo

APRIL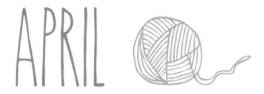

There is magic everywhere, and inside of me too. It's time for me to see it, honour it, and let it out. I am the vessel through which I express myself in the world, so how do I express my Soul? This month I give myself the opportunity to break through the blocks and barriers I put up to showing my true self to the world. I can sing, dance, write, paint or make a beautiful object or meal. I give myself my full permission. I'm excited. I do not have to share these creations with anyone if I don't want to. The Universe is asking me to create my heart's desire and I do not need to be afraid, for it already knows me in my fullness. I allow myself to be inspired by other people's art, whatever that may be, to explore and discover new things, to taste and embrace my life without fear or judgement.

EXERCISE

I close my eyes and I find myself at a tall, white, garden gate. I look at myself and I see that I am a child again. I open the gate and enter a large garden, with many playthings just waiting for me to spend time with them. What do I see? What am I drawn to? I feel the joy of a child as I skip and dance from object to object until I settle on something. There I stay and deepen my connection to it, and therefore to my own heart. I can hear humming in the background. Nature is singing to me. The Universe is alive. I am a part of it, and it is a part of me.

GOING DEEPER

Improve your skills – take a class in your chosen area of inspiration, watch YouTube and see what other people are doing, or download an app that can teach you something new. Don't be afraid to make a mistake. Everyone has to start somewhere.

THURSDAY 1

I give myself permission to live my happy life now

FRIDAY 2

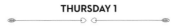

SATURDAY 3

I feel safe to experiment and make mistakes

SUNDAY 4

I am free to be myself completely

MONDAY 5

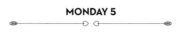

I release my need for other people's approval

TUESDAY 6

WEDNESDAY 7

I relish the sounds, smells, tastes and textures that I experience

THURSDAY 8

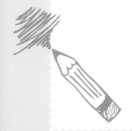

I can express myself in many different ways

FRIDAY 9

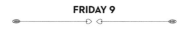

I am learning how to create a life that I love

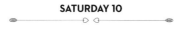

SATURDAY 10

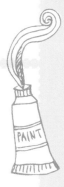

When my heart, mind and intuition are in agreement, good things happen

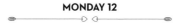

SUNDAY 11

I feel the happiness that is within me

MONDAY 12

TUESDAY 13

WEDNESDAY 14

I thank the Universe for supporting me on my healing journey

THURSDAY 15

I open my heart to love and joy and let life inspire me

FRIDAY 16

I shine my light and fill the world with love and joy

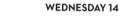

SATURDAY 17

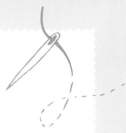

When I appreciate other people's gifts and talents, it gives me an awareness of my own

SUNDAY 18

I am patient and tolerant with myself

MONDAY 19

TUESDAY 20

I embrace the opportunities of life and I give myself permission to experience life to the full

WEDNESDAY 21

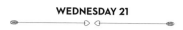

I slow down and take time to let beauty into my life

THURSDAY 22

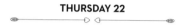

I give myself the time to do the things I need to do

FRIDAY 23

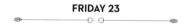

I give myself permission to follow the wisdom of my heart

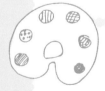

SATURDAY 24

I accept others as they are and I accept myself as I am

SUNDAY 25

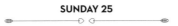

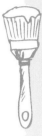

I allow my inner talent to shine through

MONDAY 26

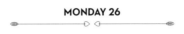

I do not need to apologise for my existence

TUESDAY 27

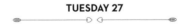

I am beautiful like me and you are beautiful like you

WEDNESDAY 28

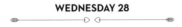

Not everything needs to be taken seriously

THURSDAY 29

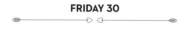

I check my energetic boundaries and expand and clear them as needed

FRIDAY 30

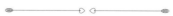

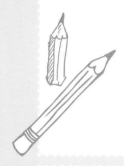

I let go of my need to get it exactly right every time

NOTES ON INSPIRATION AND CREATIVITY

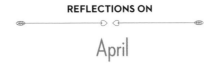

April

WHAT WAS IT LIKE TO LET YOURSELF BE TRULY CREATIVE WITHOUT BOUNDARIES? WHAT DID YOU LEARN ABOUT YOURSELF? DO YOU WANT TO CONTINUE YOUR JOURNEY INTO CREATIVITY? WHAT CAN YOU DO TO SUPPORT YOURSELF AS YOU DEEPEN YOUR CREATIVITY WITH THE THING THAT YOU LOVE?

creativity

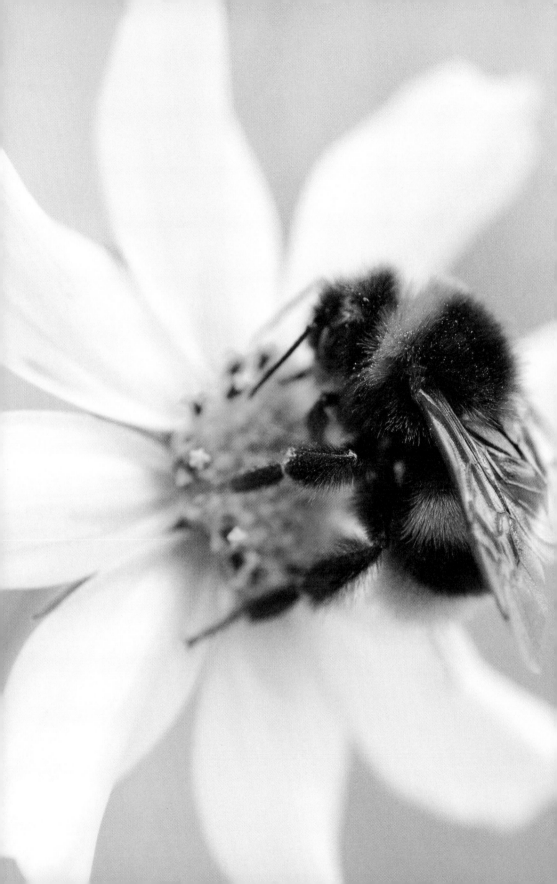

PURIFICATION AND HEALING

When I let go of all the things that are not me, I remember how good it feels to be alive.

'Where your fear is, there is your task.'

C. G. Jung

MAY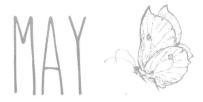

I'm taking this month to stop and audit my life. The lighter I am, the farther and higher I can fly. It's time for me to recognise what is heavy, what I am surrounded by, and what I am creating myself, so that I can let it go. It's not an easy path but it's the true and good one. They say that healing is releasing all the things that are not you, so you can begin the process of finding the truth of who you are. I want to know who I am. I give myself permission to strip away all the lies and falsehoods that I embraced to fit in, to please others or to hide myself away. I am not afraid of who I am, nor am I apologetic. I want to live lightly, authentically and truthfully, both inside and out. I will not rush this. I will take it step by step, one day at a time.

EXERCISE

I breathe and slow down. When I am feeling relaxed and connected to Mother Earth, I allow myself to visualise all the heaviness that I am carrying, as if it is contained in bags, suitcases and boxes. When I feel stabilised, I allow myself to reveal more bags to myself, as I have been hiding them the first time. I do not need to know where or what they are, I just do not need to carry them anymore. I ask Mother Earth to take away the bags that are not mine or no longer serve me. I visualise them merging into fewer bags. I see some of them dissolving away, and now I can travel light.

GOING DEEPER

You could do a detox on your space, on your physical body, or on your thoughts. Use the affirmations to help you bring your mind back to a cleaner, lighter space when a heavy thought comes in. Book a Reiki session or go to a hydrotherapy pool. Allow yourself to fully relax and let go of everything that is not yours.

SATURDAY 1

I do not need to hide anything from myself anymore

SUNDAY 2

MONDAY 3

I give myself permission to let go of emotional pain

TUESDAY 4

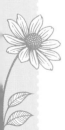

I invite healing energies to wrap themselves around me today

WEDNESDAY 5

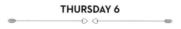

I accept others as they are, and I accept myself completely as I am

THURSDAY 6

FRIDAY 7

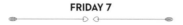

I fill myself with love so that I have love to give

SATURDAY 8

I see all my scars, my aches and pains, and it is okay

SUNDAY 9

I am doing the best that I can with what I know

MONDAY 10

Every day I heal a little bit more

TUESDAY 11

I slow down and bring my presence into the moment

WEDNESDAY 12

THURSDAY 13

I pull my energies back into my body

FRIDAY 14

I disconnect from drama and other people's expectations of me

SATURDAY 15

I am where I am and that is okay with me

SUNDAY 16

MONDAY 17

Today I will be gentle with myself

TUESDAY 18

I let go of all the things that are not me

WEDNESDAY 19

I disconnect from the ideas that I have about who I am

THURSDAY 20

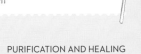

I give myself permission to be my best, healed self

FRIDAY 21

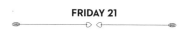

It is safe to be completely me

SATURDAY 22

I am learning how to trust myself more

SUNDAY 23

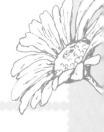

MONDAY 24

I don't always need other people's approval

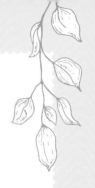

TUESDAY 25

I respect myself and only take on as much as I can handle

WEDNESDAY 26

Not everyone will like me and that's okay with me

THURSDAY 27

Today is the first day of the rest of my life

FRIDAY 28

I am compassionate and kind with myself

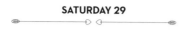

SATURDAY 29

I bring myself back to my centre and connect my feet to the ground

SUNDAY 30

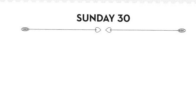

MONDAY 31

I breathe out stress and breathe in peace

NOTES ON LOVE AND HAPPINESS

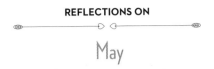
WHAT ARE YOU HAVING THE MOST DIFFICULTY IN LETTING GO? WHAT ARE YOUR BELIEFS AROUND IT?
ARE THEY TRUE? WHAT WOULD YOUR LIFE LOOK LIKE IF YOU DIDN'T BELIEVE THIS? WHAT IS IN
THE WAY OF YOU LIVING YOUR BEST AND HAPPIEST LIFE NOW? HOW CAN YOU SUPPORT
YOURSELF SO THAT YOU CAN MOVE THROUGH THIS?

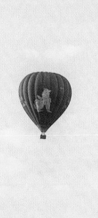

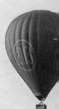

PEACE AND FORGIVENESS

Simply setting the intention to pave the way towards forgiveness puts it into motion.

'The truth is, unless you let go, unless you forgive yourself, unless you forgive the situation, unless you realize that the situation is over, you cannot move forward.'

Steve Maraboli

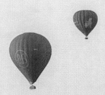

JUNE

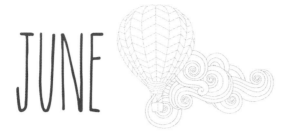

I choose to live a peaceful life. I know that peace begins with me and I have done a lot of work on myself to let go of the things that keep me from feeling peaceful. This month I commit to letting go of any anger, grudges, resentments and discontentment that I still hold inside me. This is big work, but after releasing the heaviness of last month, I can see clearly that this is also important for my healing process. When I forgive others, it frees me up to be more at peace. I want to forgive all the people in my life, including me. I do not need to forget anything. I just take the learning and move on. I separate the person out from the behaviour, and I can better understand how disempowered or upset they or I may have been at the time. I acknowledge that life is a struggle at times, and I give myself and others the benefit of the doubt.

EXERCISE

Write a list of everyone you are having difficulty with. Choose one of them and, just for a moment, put yourself in their position. Remember they see the world differently to you. Can you understand why they are taking this stance with you? You don't have to accept inappropriate behaviour. Keep your good, strong boundaries, increase the energetic space between you and them, and let go of your anger and frustration. Give them the space to be themselves, give yourself the space you need, too.

GOING DEEPER

Make a forgiveness altar and place upon it a photo of the person or people you want to forgive. You may not be ready to forgive them just yet, but by doing this you are setting your intention to become ready, in time. Spend a few minutes each day at the altar, breathing in peace and breathing out peace. Listen to your heart. Ask yourself what you need to know about the situation today. Don't be afraid to talk to a friend or get some help if you need it.

TUESDAY 1

I want to learn how to forgive myself completely

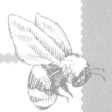

WEDNESDAY 2

THURSDAY 3

I ask for the strength that I need to let go of my anger and resentment

FRIDAY 4

I understand that I was doing the best that I could at the time

SATURDAY 5

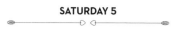

I let go of hindsight as it is not helpful to me

SUNDAY 6

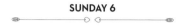

I invite healing into the part of me that is aching today

MONDAY 7

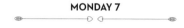

I breathe in peace and I breathe out all that is not peace

TUESDAY 8

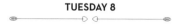

I never need to forget what happened to me, it was real and important learning

WEDNESDAY 9

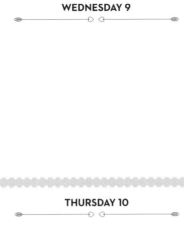

THURSDAY 10

I take my energy back from what consumes me, and I ask for it to be cleansed and healed

FRIDAY 11

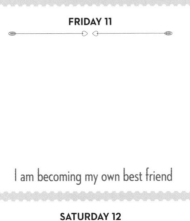

I am becoming my own best friend

SATURDAY 12

I no longer need to cause myself emotional pain

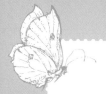

SUNDAY 13

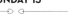

I feel safe to relax my mind and my body

MONDAY 14

I bring my awareness back to the present moment

TUESDAY 15

I slow down and connect to my heart

WEDNESDAY 16

THURSDAY 17

I am grateful for all my relationships and the learning they have brought me

FRIDAY 18

I can have good, strong boundaries and maintain healthy relationships

SATURDAY 19

I am able to say the things I need to say

SUNDAY 20

I give myself permission to release anything that is not peace

MONDAY 21

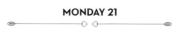

I choose to fill my world with peace and love

TUESDAY 22

I disconnect from fear and anger and I choose love

WEDNESDAY 23

THURSDAY 24

Please show me what I need to do today so that I can be at peace

FRIDAY 25

I can say no with love in my heart

SATURDAY 26

SUNDAY 27

I am kind and compassionate towards myself

MONDAY 28

I allow myself to be at peace with myself

TUESDAY 29

Today I choose peace over fear

WEDNESDAY 30

I start and end my day with peace

NOTES ON PEACE AND FORGIVENESS

June

HOW ARE YOU FEELING AFTER DOING THE WORK OF THIS MONTH? WHO OR WHAT DO YOU STILL HAVE TO FORGIVE? WHAT IS IT THAT YOU ARE EXPECTING OR THAT IS HOLDING YOU BACK?

These past few months, we experienced themes of Inspiration and Creativity, Purification and Healing, Peace and Forgiveness. You have done a lot of work, some of it very deep, which will have long-lasting effects on your life.

Take some time right now to sit with all that you have learned and all that you feel you have achieved. Well done.

WHAT DO YOU FEEL WAS YOUR GREATEST MOMENT OF THE PAST THREE MONTHS?

WHAT WAS THE MOST DIFFICULT? HOW DID YOU LOOK AFTER YOURSELF IN IT?

HOW DO YOU PLAN TO MOVE FORWARD AND EMBODY ALL THAT YOU HAVE LEARNED?

_____

_____

_____

_____

GO BACK THROUGH THE DIARY AND CHOOSE YOUR FAVOURITE AFFIRMATION, ONE FROM THE PAST THREE MONTHS THAT MADE THE MOST DIFFERENCE TO YOU. WRITE IT DOWN HERE FOR SAFEKEEPING.

_____

_____

_____

_____

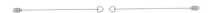

Go to my website, www.abby-wynne.com/onedayatatime, and make sure you have signed up for my bonus recordings. Perhaps you'd like to take some time to listen to a few of the visualisations and meditations to consolidate what you have done so far this year.

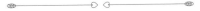

Now we move to the next three months of the year. If you are still doing the work of the last three months, know that you must do your healing at your own pace. Don't forget that you can revisit any of the affirmations and exercises of the past three months and bring them with you as additional support.

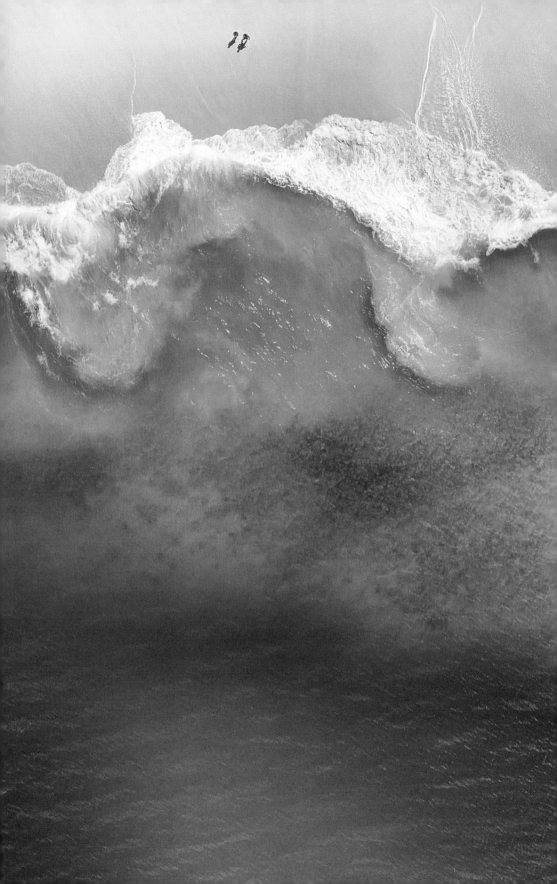

AUTHENTICITY AND VITALITY

The more authentic I am,
the brighter my inner light shines.

'When someone tells me no, it doesn't mean I can't do it,
it simply means I can't do it with them.'

Karen E. Quinones Miller

JULY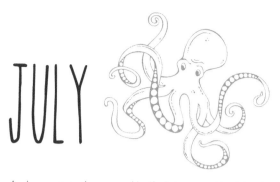

As I move into the second half of the year, I look back at all I've learned. I'm taking better care of myself and I'm happier for it. I'm working on forgiving everyone, including myself. I feel lighter and stronger. I've allowed myself to express myself creatively and be inspired by beauty and joy. I've let go of the burden of heaviness that I carried for far too long. I feel free, and I like who I am becoming. I know it can be a risk to show myself to others, but I'm learning that the cost of not doing so weighs more heavily upon me than it did before. This month I want to bring together everything I've learned, and access my inner zest for life. I feel nature's life force energy around me. I want to add to it instead of hiding away. I sleep better at night. I trust myself more. I am no longer afraid of who I am.

EXERCISE

Slow down and breathe. Close your eyes and visualise a clear, bright, white light, strong and beautiful, entering the place where you are and settling over your head. This ball of light is filled with healing and vitality. Feel it entering your head, moving slowly down and into all the parts of your body, filling them up with light. It rests in your heart centre and shines out from you, filling the room with light, the city with light, the country with light. You are the light.

GOING DEEPER

Start telling people how you really feel. Stop saying sorry when you are not really sorry. Find other ways to say what you mean to say. Do what you say you are going to do. Say no to things that you are not able to do. Enjoy the energy and lightness of living in truth.

THURSDAY 1

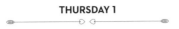

I am becoming someone who I would trust with my own life

FRIDAY 2

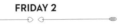

SATURDAY 3

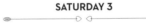

I am no longer apologetic for who I am

SUNDAY 4

I can agree to disagree with someone and still remain friends

MONDAY 5

I take a step back from the situation and reconnect to me

TUESDAY 6

WEDNESDAY 7

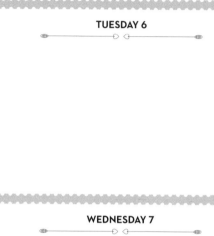

I shine my bright light out into the world

THURSDAY 8

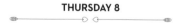

I am proud of how far I have come on my healing journey

FRIDAY 9

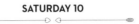

I ask for all my energy to come back to me

SATURDAY 10

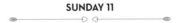

I love being alive today

SUNDAY 11

I love being alive today

I see all the opportunities in everything

MONDAY 12

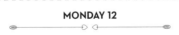

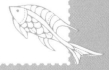

Today I see all the opportunities in everything

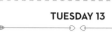

TUESDAY 13

I am grateful for the sun that shines, even when it is behind a cloud

WEDNESDAY 14

I connect to Mother Earth, I am grounded

THURSDAY 15

It feels so good to be free, to be real, to speak my truth

FRIDAY 16

SATURDAY 17

I speak up and can say what I need to say without fear

SUNDAY 18

All is as it should be

MONDAY 19

I am doing better every day

TUESDAY 20

I invite healing energies to pour into me and out through me

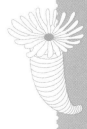

WEDNESDAY 21

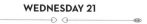

I am not afraid to be excited and learn new things

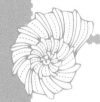

THURSDAY 22

I invite joy and love into my life

FRIDAY 23

I trust the Universe is looking after me in perfect ways

SATURDAY 24

I am grateful for my body and the work it does for me in the background

SUNDAY 25

I can see the beauty in everything

MONDAY 26

TUESDAY 27

I am learning how to love myself more

WEDNESDAY 28

I look forward to what the day may bring

THURSDAY 29

Love softens all my hard edges

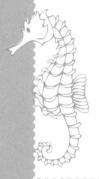

FRIDAY 30

SATURDAY 31

I shine my light out to the world and see love reflected back in everything

NOTES ON AUTHENTICITY AND VITALITY

HOW DID YOU GET ON WITH THE EXERCISE OF BEING TRUTHFUL? DID YOU MANAGE TO GO DEEPER?
WHAT WAS THAT LIKE FOR YOU?

WHERE DID YOU GET STUCK? WHAT WILL YOU DO NEXT TIME YOU GET STUCK IN A SIMILAR WAY?
CAN YOU STILL FORGIVE YOURSELF COMPLETELY?

AUTHENTICITY AND VITALITY

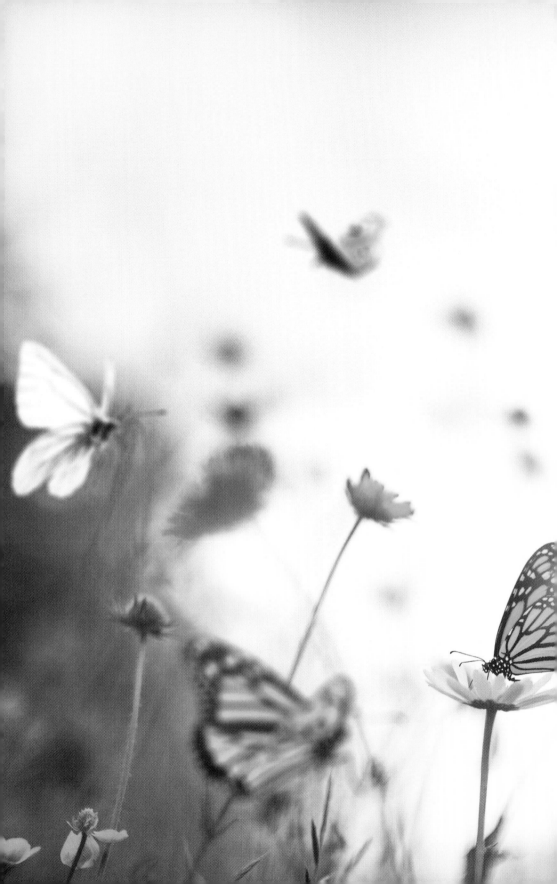

PRESENCE AND BEAUTY

When I slow down and come into the present moment, I see the beauty that has always been here.

'If you want your life to have depth and meaning, be present, be mindful, and live with intention.'

Akiroq Brost

AUGUST

The world is an amazing place, always changing, always in motion. As am I – growing and changing moment to moment. This month I will slow down and appreciate the beauty in all things. I allow myself to sit in stillness and I can be with difficult emotions as well as wonderful ones. I let them all flow through me because they are not me. I am the mountain and they are the weather, and they will eventually pass me by. I am coming into alignment with myself and the world. It is easier to be at peace and to be fully present in the moment. I have more compassion and I can see the beauty in all living things. I appreciate my life more and more and I want to invite more beauty into my life, every day.

EXERCISE

I take time with my cup of tea and sit in stillness. I bring my presence inwards, to my body, and focus my awareness on my face. What is going on for me? I ask my mind to tell me everything that is troubling it. I listen with compassion and make note of it. I then bring my awareness to my heart, doing the same thing, and finally to my stomach, where I do it once more. I am here, with myself, and I can look after myself. Everything will be okay.

GOING DEEPER

Recognise your own beauty – the beauty of experiencing emotions, the beauty of love and connection. Bring more beauty into your day. Buy yourself flowers, get a new perfume or scented candle. Spend some time with beauty, really admiring it. What is beautiful for you?

SUNDAY 1
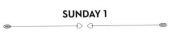

There is great beauty in small things

MONDAY 2
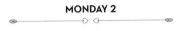

I step away from my thoughts and feelings and take the time to see what is actually here

TUESDAY 3
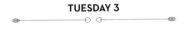

I choose to fill my world with peace and love

WEDNESDAY 4
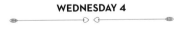

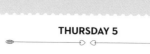

THURSDAY 5

I connect to my intuition and listen to my inner wisdom

FRIDAY 6

I bring myself back to my centre and feel my feet on the ground

SATURDAY 7

I can find beauty in ordinary things

SUNDAY 8

I slow down and bring my awareness into the present moment

MONDAY 9

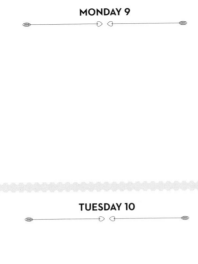

TUESDAY 10

I relish the smells, sounds, colours and tastes that I experience

WEDNESDAY 11

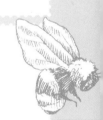

When I make space for myself, I have more space for other people

THURSDAY 12

I sit down and relax and bring myself back to the present moment

FRIDAY 13

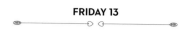

There can be beauty in difficult situations

SATURDAY 14

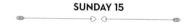

I give myself permission to let more beauty into my life

SUNDAY 15

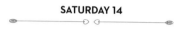

I feel safe to let go of things that no longer bring me joy

MONDAY 16

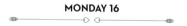

TUESDAY 17

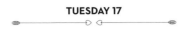

When I open to beauty, I feel alive and present in the world

WEDNESDAY 18

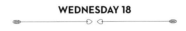

I breathe in beauty and breathe out all that is not beauty

THURSDAY 19

I allow life to surprise me with beauty in unexpected places

FRIDAY 20

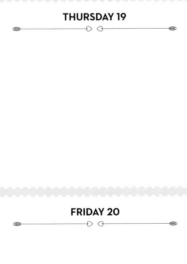

SATURDAY 21

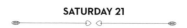

I am safe, I am centred, I am grounded, I am here

SUNDAY 22

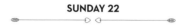

I let go of all my worries and bring myself into the present moment

MONDAY 23

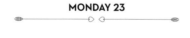

TUESDAY 24

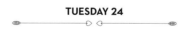

I step away from heaviness and find myself again

WEDNESDAY 25

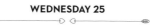

I am learning how to enjoy the good things in life

THURSDAY 26

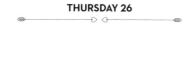

FRIDAY 27

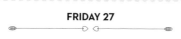

I am grateful that I live a life filled with joy, hope and inspiration

SATURDAY 28

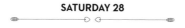

I deliberately choose to bring more beauty into my life

SUNDAY 29

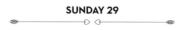

When I fill my heart with love, I resonate with beauty and joy

MONDAY 30

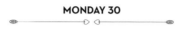

I leave a trail of love behind me

TUESDAY 31

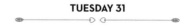

Today I will be slow and gentle with myself

NOTES ON PRESENCE AND BEAUTY

August

WHAT DIFFERENCES CAN YOU FEEL IN YOUR BODY WHEN YOU'RE PRESENT AND WHEN YOU'RE NOT? WHAT CAN YOU USE AS AN INDICATOR TO HELP KEEP YOU MORE PRESENT IN THE MOMENT?

HOW DID YOU BRING BEAUTY INTO YOUR LIFE THIS MONTH? WHAT WOULD YOU LIKE TO INVITE INTO YOUR LIFE NEXT MONTH?

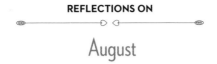

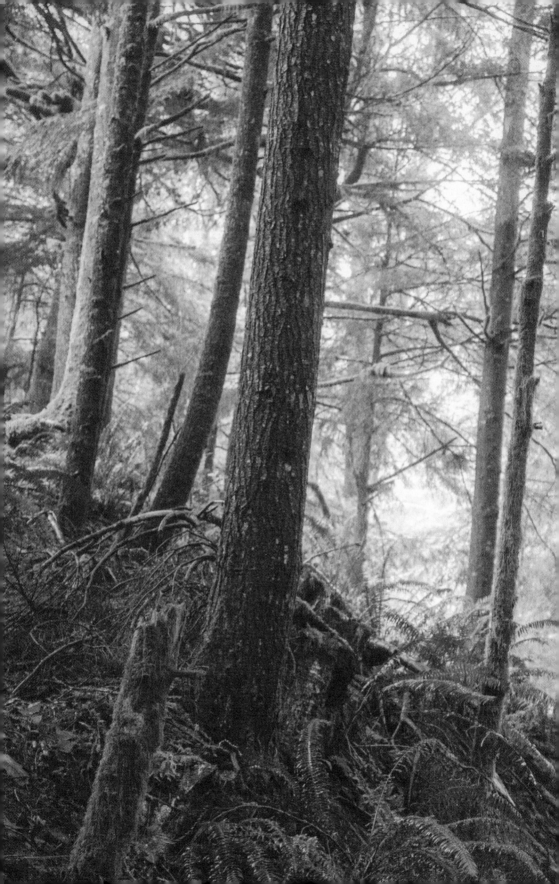

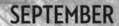

SAFETY AND GROUNDING

**I am here, I am safe.
Everything is as it should be.**

'Feeling rooted in the earth is soothing to the body,
and it is our connection to the earth that gives us our most
basic sense of belonging, home, resilience, and safety.'

Jessica Moore

SEPTEMBER

This month the energies are intense. I will pull back and focus on staying grounded and feeling safe. As I do my inner work I allow for the release of patterns and old emotions. I know that I am always in a process of healing. I can do this in my own time, in my own way. I do not need to rush anything. I allow myself to take days off and get additional rest if needed. I give myself permission to simply get through the day, and that is enough. I let go of my expectations and come back to the basics, breathing through waves of anxiety if they come. I can simplify my life and enjoy the small things – the taste of food, the company of a good friend, or a book or movie that I love. I do not need to engage with fear. I switch off the news and spend time in nature instead. I know the sun sets and rises, and tomorrow is another day.

EXERCISE

I lie down on the ground and breathe and soften my body. I feel the earth beneath me, holding me completely. I slow down my breath, I slow down my thoughts, and I bring myself more deeply inwards. I am here, I am safe. I am here, I am safe. I repeat my mantra and I feel centred and contained. I repeat my mantra to each part of my body until I feel at peace.

GOING DEEPER

Notice your high expectations of yourself. What do you think you should be doing? Write them down. Are they realistic? Ask yourself why you're holding yourself to them so tightly, and then let them go. What if you get more done this month by being still, instead of being active?

WEDNESDAY 1

I drop an anchor from my body into Mother Earth and I feel secure

THURSDAY 2

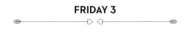

I feel my feet on the ground and bring myself into the present moment

FRIDAY 3

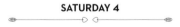

I give myself permission to relax

SATURDAY 4

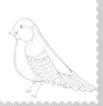

SUNDAY 5

There will be time to do the things I need to do

MONDAY 6

I allow myself to look after myself

TUESDAY 7

It is safe to experience all of my emotions

WEDNESDAY 8

I am more peaceful when I am compassionate and patient towards myself

THURSDAY 9

FRIDAY 10

I walk away from drama and choose peace instead

SATURDAY 11

I slow down and connect to my heart

SUNDAY 12

I am grateful for my body and how much work it does for me in the background

MONDAY 13

I am learning how to accept all parts of myself

TUESDAY 14

I use my breath to slow down my thoughts

WEDNESDAY 15

I no longer need to struggle with myself

THURSDAY 16

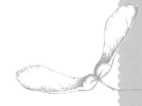

FRIDAY 17

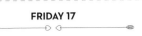

I feel the earth beneath my feet, I am here, I am safe

SATURDAY 18

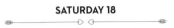

I grow deep roots like the oldest trees and feel held

SUNDAY 19

I expand my energy and relax; there is no need to push or force anything

MONDAY 20

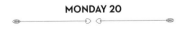

I check my anchor and make it stronger and deeper

TUESDAY 21

Today I will wrap myself in love

WEDNESDAY 22

I breathe in love and breathe out all that is not love

THURSDAY 23

I choose love over fear

FRIDAY 24

Today I will give everyone the benefit of the doubt

SATURDAY 25

I am safe, I am strong, I am here

SUNDAY 26

MONDAY 27

I am able to live a life full of love

TUESDAY 28

I am loving and kind to myself and to others

WEDNESDAY 29

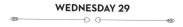

I bring patience and love into everything that I do

THURSDAY 30

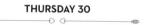

NOTES ON SAFETY AND GROUNDING

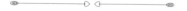

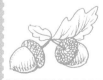

September

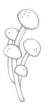

WHAT WAS YOUR BIGGEST LEARNING THIS MONTH?

WHAT DO YOU LIKE TO DO TO SUPPORT YOURSELF WHEN YOU'RE FRAGILE?

During the past few months we experienced themes
of Authenticity and Vitality, Presence and Beauty,
Safety and Grounding. These are all big, strong themes.
Which one affected you the most?

Do you feel you're able to look after yourself better,
based on the learning that you've already gained this year?

WHAT DO YOU FEEL WAS YOUR GREATEST MOMENT OF THE PAST THREE MONTHS?

_____

_____

_____

_____

_____

WHAT WAS THE MOST DIFFICULT? HOW DID YOU LOOK AFTER YOURSELF IN IT?

_____

_____

_____

_____

_____

HOW DO YOU PLAN TO MOVE FORWARD AND EMBODY ALL THAT YOU HAVE LEARNED?

GO BACK THROUGH THE DIARY AND CHOOSE YOUR FAVOURITE AFFIRMATION, ONE FROM THE PAST THREE MONTHS THAT MADE THE MOST DIFFERENCE TO YOU. WRITE IT DOWN HERE FOR SAFEKEEPING.

Go to my website, www.abby-wynne.com/onedayatatime, and make sure you have signed up for my bonus recordings. Perhaps you'd like to take some time to listen to a few of the visualisations and meditations to consolidate what you have done so far this year.

Now we move to the next three months of the year. If you are still doing the work of the last three months, know that you must do your healing at your own pace. Don't forget that you can revisit any of the affirmations and exercises of the past three months and bring them with you as additional support.

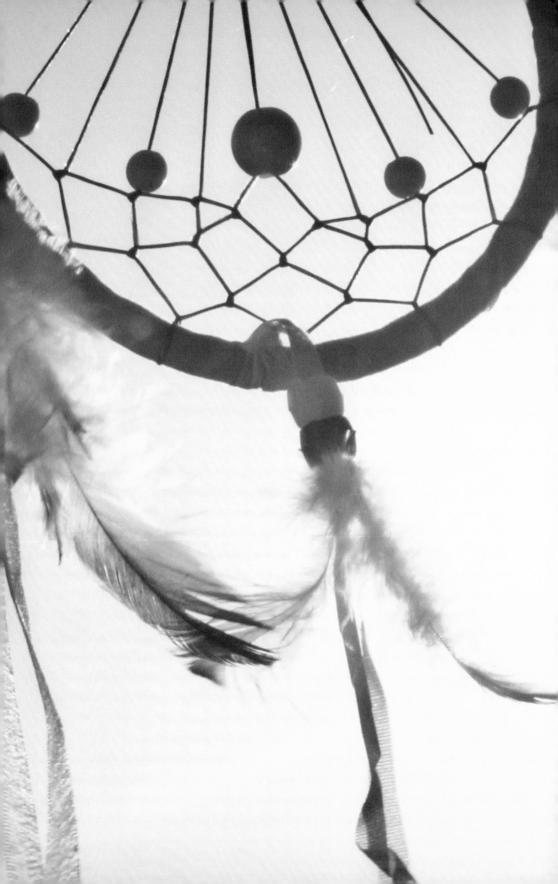

OCTOBER

BALANCE AND STABILITY

**I am ready for my happy life now.
I no longer need to sabotage my growth process.**

'They who reach down into the depths of life where, in the stillness,
the voice of God is heard, have the stabilising power which carries
them poised and serene through the hurricane of difficulties.'

Spencer W. Kimball

OCTOBER

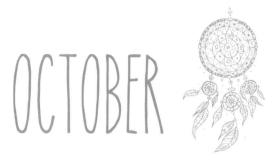

As I find my footing, I realise that I am stronger and more confident than I've ever been in my life. I choose to be happy, to abandon the old scripts where I was critical and mean to myself, to let go of old patterns of sabotage. Life is precious and more valuable than I realised. I will not waste any more of it holding myself back. This month I will come into balance with the idea that I no longer need to cause myself emotional pain. I give myself permission to blossom and exist. Things happen around me and not to me. I do not need to take them personally. Everyone is experiencing their own growth process. I can see the person beneath the behaviours and the messiness of life, and I love them regardless. I deliberately choose love over fear, fun and joy over misery, and I allow myself to experience all of my emotions.

EXERCISE

I feel my feet on the ground. I grow roots down deep through the rocks and stones and into Mother Earth until I feel solid and strong. I grow to my full energetic size. Then I expand to bigger than I realise. I am bigger than the house, bigger than the street or the town where I live. I breathe in light and I breathe out fear. I am stable, I am balanced, I am here.

GOING DEEPER

Do the exercise once a day for a week and see how you feel by the end of it. When you are expanded, visualise ropes of fear that are holding you back. Notice what they are tied to, and then give yourself permission to cut them away.

FRIDAY 1

I let go of my ideal self and I embrace who I am today

SATURDAY 2

I allow myself to make mistakes and to grow

SUNDAY 3

I am proud of how far I have come

MONDAY 4

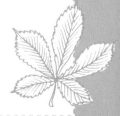

TUESDAY 5

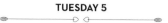

I am learning how to look after me

WEDNESDAY 6

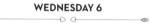

Every day I love myself a little bit more

THURSDAY 7

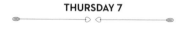

I connect to a source of unconditional love and feel it ripple through my body

FRIDAY 8

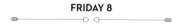

I expand my energies and I remember who I am

SATURDAY 9

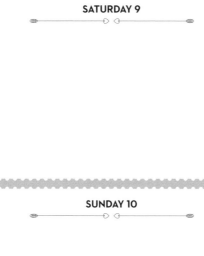

SUNDAY 10

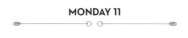

I am not afraid to speak what is true for me

MONDAY 11

I am free to be completely myself in this moment

TUESDAY 12

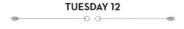

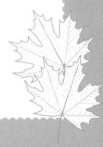

I allow myself to enjoy the beauty in the world

WEDNESDAY 13

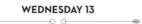

I can sit in stillness with my thoughts and emotions and not be overwhelmed

THURSDAY 14

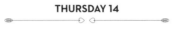

My heart is filled with compassion towards myself and others

FRIDAY 15

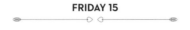

When my inner light shines bright it reminds others they can shine theirs too

SATURDAY 16

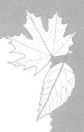

SUNDAY 17

I give myself permission to relax

MONDAY 18

I let go of fear and choose everything from a place of love

TUESDAY 19

I accept myself completely just as I am

WEDNESDAY 20

I make time to do everything I need to do

THURSDAY 21

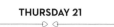

I listen to my body and give it what it needs

FRIDAY 22

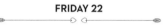

I am grateful for all my relationships

SATURDAY 23

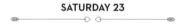

SUNDAY 24

I deliberately surround myself with things that lift my spirits

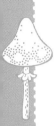

MONDAY 25

I invite more happiness and joy into my life

TUESDAY 26

WEDNESDAY 27

I allow myself to show up for life

THURSDAY 28

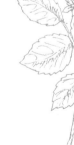

I am not afraid to be in vibrant health

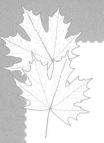

FRIDAY 29

SATURDAY 30

I make space to process and heal

SUNDAY 31

NOTES ON BALANCE AND STABILITY

OCTOBER

October

WHEN YOU ARE YOUR BEST, HEALED SELF, YOU ALLOW YOURSELF TO EXPERIENCE YOUR EMOTIONS AND YOU GIVE YOURSELF TIME TO PROCESS AND HEAL. WHAT DO YOU NEED TO DO TO COME INTO BALANCE WITH THIS STATEMENT?

WHAT DAILY PRACTICES CAN YOU BEGIN TO INCORPORATE INTO YOUR LIFE THAT WILL HELP YOU FEEL EMOTIONALLY STABLE?

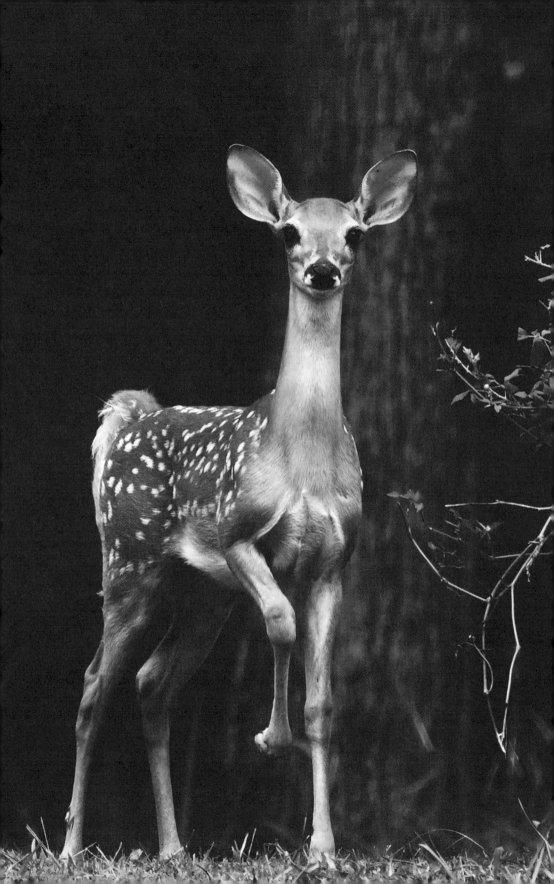

RESILIENCE AND GRACE

Grace is divine life-force energy.
I feel it strongly in me
and I see it everywhere.

'If your heart is broken, make art with the pieces.'

Shane Koyczan

NOVEMBER

Love is stronger than fear. Love will always win, and more and more I find myself choosing from love. With love in my heart I know I will prevail. I have survived my life up to this moment and now I want to thrive. Life is beautiful. I see the wonder and grace of the miracle of everything. A newborn baby; a beautiful flower; the way the flames flicker in the fire; the light behind someone's eyes when they smile. There is such beauty here. How could I have missed so much of it? Even in the mundane and ordinary things there is grace. I am grateful to have this opportunity to be alive, to know myself, to feel consolidated and strong. I see myself standing up to my full height, offering my creations to the world. With love and grace in my heart, I can be a beacon of light.

EXERCISE

I close my eyes, breathe and relax, and let go of my need to fix or change anything. I connect to my heartbeat and I can hear my breath. I can feel life pulsing though my body and my nervous system. I feel the flow of life within me. I feel my divine life-force energy and I recognise it in everything around me. I imagine that I stand up tall and that love shines outwards from my heart until I become a lighthouse guiding everyone home.

GOING DEEPER

Recognise when you revert back to your old survival patterns and congratulate yourself for being here now. Start to create a new pattern for thriving. Ask yourself what that would look like. Write it down. Make it real. Start putting it into practice.

MONDAY 1

Today I will shine my bright, inner light outwards to the world

TUESDAY 2

WEDNESDAY 3

I do not need to fix or change anyone else

THURSDAY 4

I am becoming the master of my thoughts and emotions

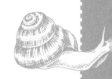

I spend time in silence and connect to a source of love

I do not need to run from myself anymore

I am not afraid of my emotions

I am not afraid of my thoughts

TUESDAY 9

I choose to invest in myself

WEDNESDAY 10

I am worthy of love

THURSDAY 11

FRIDAY 12

I am grateful for the small details of my day

SATURDAY 13

I allow myself to feel happy today

SUNDAY 14

I do not need to take things personally

MONDAY 15

I will never abandon myself

TUESDAY 16

WEDNESDAY 17

I can give myself everything I need

THURSDAY 18

I am filled with joy and appreciation for everything in my life

FRIDAY 19

I can see the beauty in everything

SATURDAY 20

My day starts with love and ends with love

SUNDAY 21

I accept myself completely for who I am

MONDAY 22

I trust that everything is as it should be

TUESDAY 23

I hand my troubles over to the Universe and I feel the burden lifting off me

WEDNESDAY 24

I let go of my need to always be right

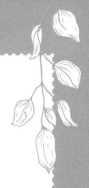

THURSDAY 25

When I am at peace, I stop struggling with life

FRIDAY 26

SATURDAY 27

I slow down and reconnect to my heart

SUNDAY 28

I choose to find the peace and beauty in everything

MONDAY 29

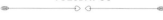

I trust that the Universe is looking after me in perfect ways

TUESDAY 30

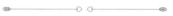

NOTES ON RESILIENCE AND GRACE

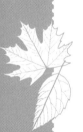

WHAT DOES GRACE MEAN TO YOU? HOW CAN YOU SPEND MORE
TIME CONNECTING TO A SOURCE OF GRACE?

HOW HAVE YOU MOVED PAST YOUR OLD SCRIPTS AND BEHAVIOURS THIS MONTH? WHAT DID YOU DO
THAT YOU WOULDN'T HAVE DONE BEFORE? HOW DID THAT MAKE YOU FEEL?

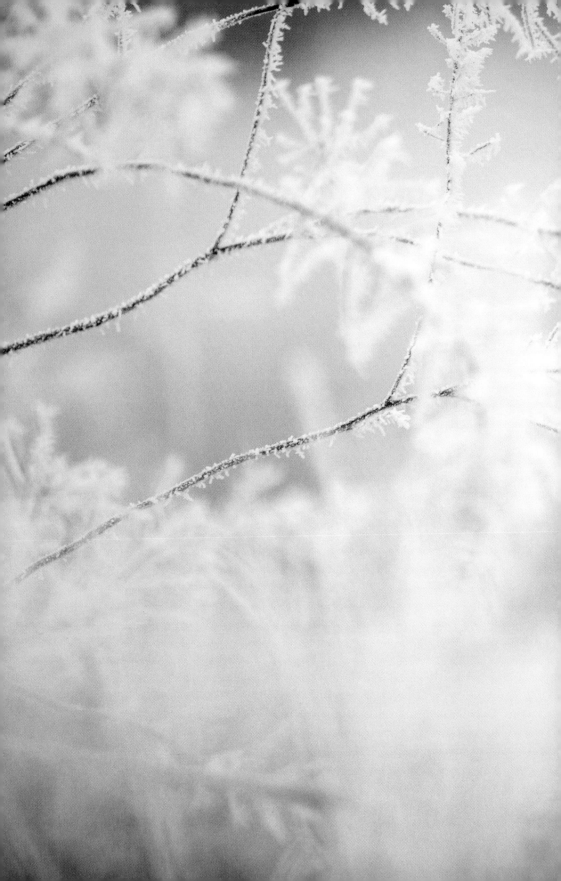

DECEMBER

LOVE AND GRATITUDE

Healing is happening all the time,
in layers and in levels. I let the love in,
and I am excited and grateful for
where my journey brings me.

'Expectation has brought me disappointment.
Disappointment has brought me wisdom.
Acceptance, gratitude and appreciation have
brought me joy and fulfilment.'

Rasheed Ogunlaru

DECEMBER

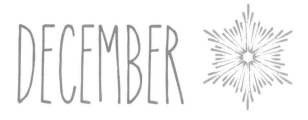

It is the end of the year. I look back on all its highs and its lows, and I look deeper at myself and the person that I am becoming. I can say with grace in my heart that I like myself more. I am better able to take care of myself. I have more patience and tolerance for others and for myself. I have done my forgiveness work, I am learning how to express myself creatively without fear, and I stand in a place of love. I am authentic in word and deed, and I love how much freedom being truthful gives me. I still have bad days and wobbly moments, but I am able to support myself through them. I trust myself at a deeper level and I am more confident listening to my inner voice. I see now that I do not have to force or push through a block. I can sit and honour myself and bring in love.

EXERCISE

I sit in silence and breathe. I bring my awareness inwards. I start at my feet. Hello, feet, I am grateful for all the work that you do for me. Thank you. I love you. I move to my ankles. Hello, ankles, I am grateful to you for keeping me upright and straight. Thank you. I love you. Continue this exercise and speak to all your body parts. Be authentic and only say what is true for you, always ending with 'thank you, I love you'. Notice how you feel afterwards.

GOING DEEPER

Take the exercise outside to nature or try it in the bath or the car. Keep saying 'thank you, I love you' in your mind. Find some music that lifts you and sing it. Make it a mantra for your life.

WEDNESDAY 1

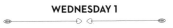

I give permission for my heart to heal

THURSDAY 2

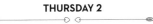

FRIDAY 3

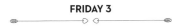

I slow down and can feel the love that is around me

SATURDAY 4

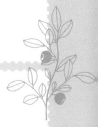

Everything I do I do with love

SUNDAY 5

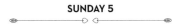

I release my need and expectations and return to a source of love

MONDAY 6

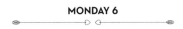

Thank you, I love you; thank you, I love you

TUESDAY 7

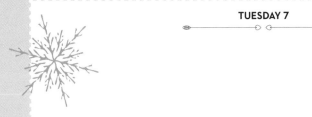

I vibrate at the frequency of love

WEDNESDAY 8

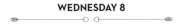

I accept myself completely as I am

THURSDAY 9

FRIDAY 10

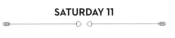

I am grateful to be in the flow of life

SATURDAY 11

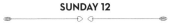

It is safe to give and receive love

SUNDAY 12

I release the blocks that I have to love

MONDAY 13

TUESDAY 14

Everywhere I see miracles around me

WEDNESDAY 15

I am grateful for my happy life now

THURSDAY 16

I respect myself and see how far I have come

FRIDAY 17

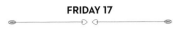

I open my heart and receive the love that is here for me

SATURDAY 18

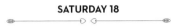

I am grateful to live a life filled with hope, joy and inspiration

SUNDAY 19

I am patient and kind with myself and others

MONDAY 20

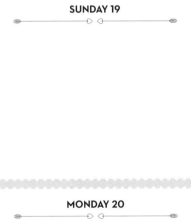

I am patient and kind with myself and others

TUESDAY 21

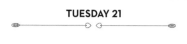

I let life inspire me

WEDNESDAY 22

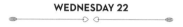

I respect all human beings no matter where they are on their journey

THURSDAY 23

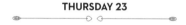

I start my day and end my day with gratitude, grace and love

FRIDAY 24

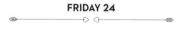

When I am centred in the present moment, I can choose from a place of love

SATURDAY 25
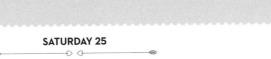

Today I let go of my resistance to love

SUNDAY 26
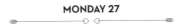

MONDAY 27
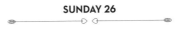

I am grateful for all the beauty in my life

TUESDAY 28
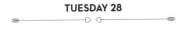

I am thankful for the lessons that I have learned and am still learning

WEDNESDAY 29

I trust myself to look after myself well

THURSDAY 30

FRIDAY 31

I love who I am becoming

NOTES ON LOVE AND GRATITUDE

DECEMBER

December

WHAT WAS IT LIKE FOR YOU TO FOCUS COMPLETELY ON LOVE? WHAT DID YOU FIND DIFFICULT ABOUT
IT? WHAT DID YOU LIKE BEST?

HOW CAN YOU LOOK AFTER YOURSELF DURING THE HOLIDAYS AND INTO THE COMING YEAR?

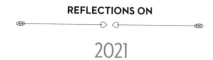

2021

The last three themes were Balance and Stability, Resilience and Grace, Love and Gratitude. What was it like for you to move from difficult energies into high vibrational grace, love and gratitude? Did you feel any differences in your body? How are you feeling now?

Take some time right now to sit with all that you have learned, and all that you feel you have achieved. Well done.

WHAT DO YOU FEEL WAS YOUR GREATEST MOMENT OF THE YEAR?

WHAT WAS THE MOST DIFFICULT? HOW DID YOU LOOK AFTER YOURSELF?

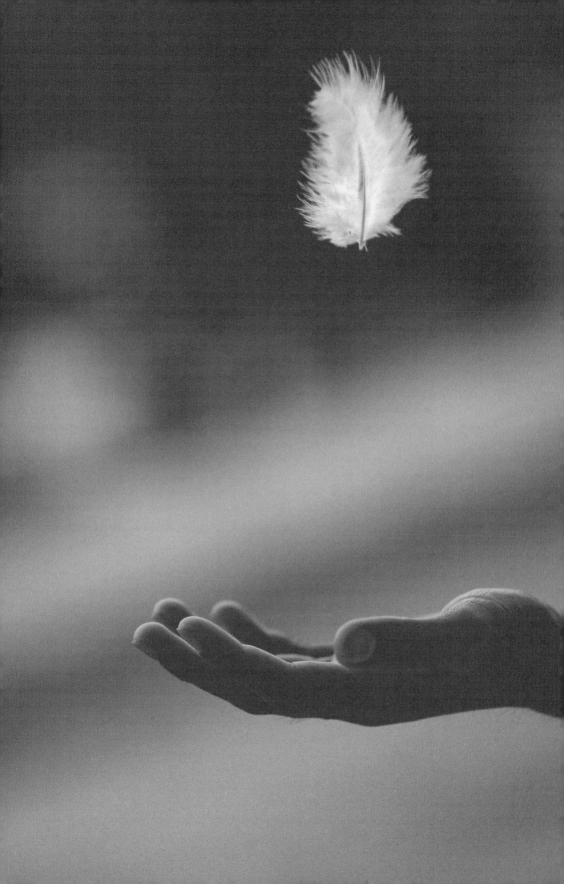

2021

WHAT WOULD YOU WISH FOR YOURSELF FOR 2022? WHAT NEW SKILLS COULD YOU BRING INTO YOUR LIFE? DO YOU HAVE PLANS TO TRAVEL MORE OR DEVELOP NEW RELATIONSHIPS?

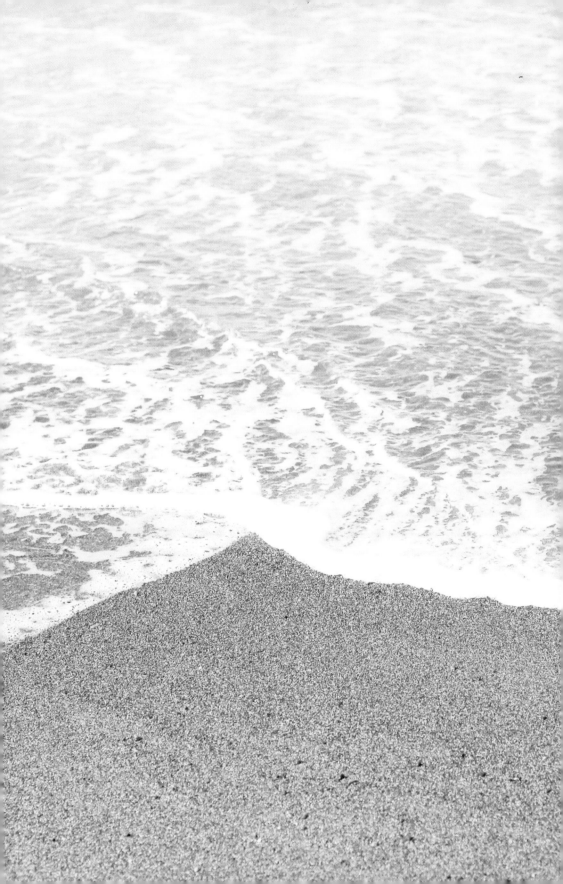

ACKNOWLEDGEMENTS

Huge thanks once again to Lorna Bevan for her consultation work, which helped establish the themes in this year's diary. I believe that her input has made this diary more dynamic and, therefore, more useful to readers. You can find her at www.hareinthemoonastrology.co.uk.

Gratitude to Sarah Liddy, commissioning editor and co-creator at Gill Books, and to Jane Matthews, designer supreme, for her beautiful design that melds my words with the images so perfectly. I also want to thank everyone at Gill Books, who work hard behind the scenes to get yet another fabulous diary into the world.

Finally, thanks to my family, particularly to my husband, Ian, for understanding me, being patient with me, and giving me all the space that I need to grow.